5 Steps to
Healthy Nutrition

Learn about

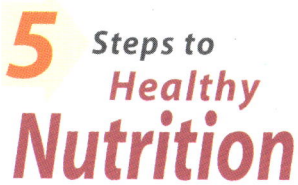

5 Steps to *Healthy* Nutrition

Dr. ANJALI ARORA

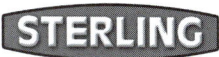

STERLING PAPERBACKS
An imprint of
Sterling Publishers (P) Ltd.
Regd. Office: A-59, Okhla Industrial Area, Phase-II,
New Delhi-110020. CIN: U22110PB1964PTC002569
Tel: 26387070, 26386209; Fax: 91-11-26383788
E-mail: mail@sterlingpublishers.com
www.sterlingpublishers.com

5 Steps to
Healthy Nutrition
© 2007, *Dr. Anjali Arora*
arora_doc@hotmail.com
ISBN 978 81 207 3248 3
Reprint 2008, 2009, 2010, 2011, 2012, 2013, 2014

The author wishes to thank all academicians, scientists and writers who have been a source of inspiration.

The author and publisher specifically disclaim any liability, loss or risk, whatsoever, personal or otherwise, which is incurred as a consequence, directly or indirectly of the use and application of any of the contents of this book.

All rights are reserved.
No part of this publication may be reproduced, stored in a retrieval system or transmitted, in any form or by any means, mechanical, photocopying, recording or otherwise, without prior written permission of the authors.

Printed and Published by Sterling Publishers Pvt. Ltd., New Delhi-110020.

Contents

1. Understanding Your Diet — 8
2. Food Blocks — 10
3. Keep Your Palate Under Control — 39
4. A Healthy Meal Plan — 46
5. Food Labels and Good Nutrition — 58
   Myths and Fact File — 63

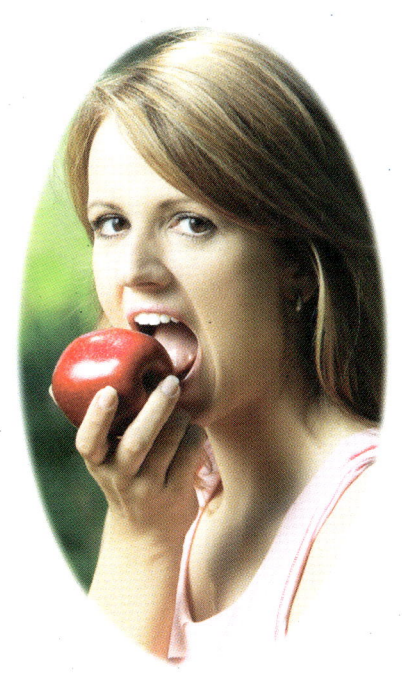

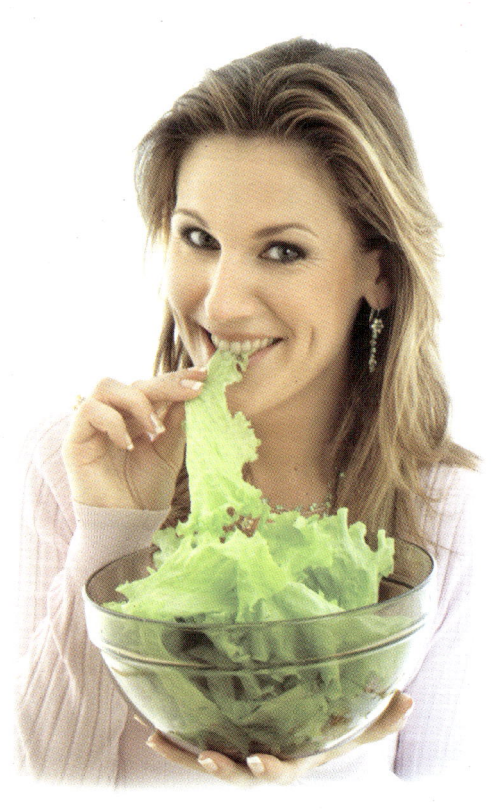

The joy of knowing what you can eat comes through a clear idea of the kinds of foods one can consume. And there is such a variety. A lot has been said about fats, high cholesterol, carbohydrates and proteins. But what are they? Why is it so important to know about each of them? You should be familiar with your foods in order to decide what exactly is needed by your body. How healthy is it for you at your age to have more of one type of a food block and less of the other. Give yourself the pleasure of juggling and deciding as to what your diet should be.

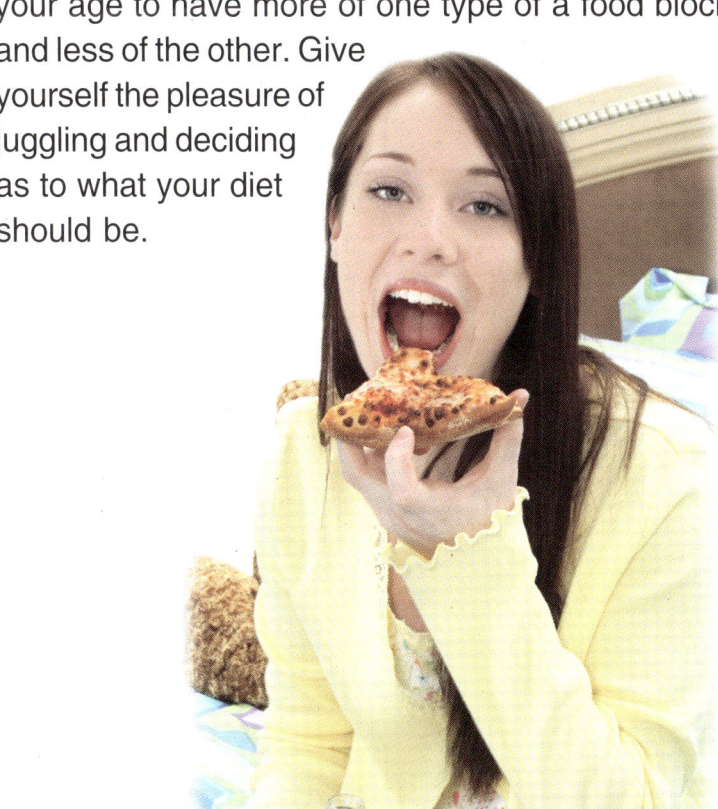

1 Understanding Your Diet

The Sweet Tooth

- Do you eat desserts, puddings or ice creams at least three times a week.
- You do not consume fruit with each main meal.

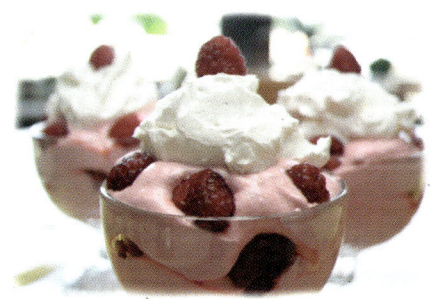

Rich food

- Do you eat out at least three times a week.
- While eating out you enjoy food rich in butter, cheese, rich stuffing, etc.

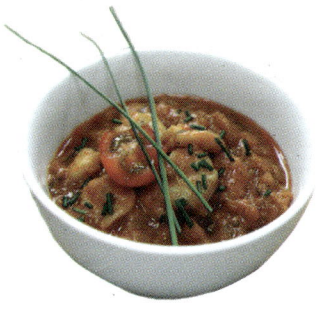

Alcohol

- Do you drink alcohol 3-4 times a week.
- Do you consume more than 60 ml of whisky, gin, rum (hard drink) or more than 2 glasses of wine each day.

Snacking

- Do you like to snack on fried food items with your drink.
- Do you enjoy sweets, packaged or fried snack with tea.

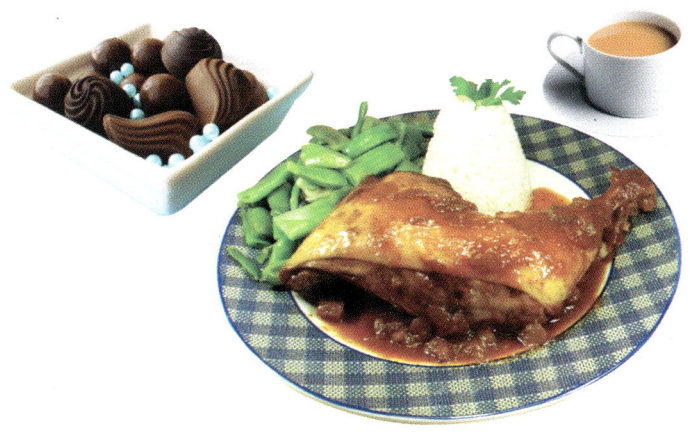

The more times you answer yes, the more is your consumption of unhealthy food throughout the day.

2   *Food Blocks*

Foods are the nourishers of our body, mind, moods and soul. Have you noticed that they even give us pleasure? All types of diet are being advocated – South beach diet, Pritkins diet, Atkins diet and so on. Some individuals may have been helped through some of these.

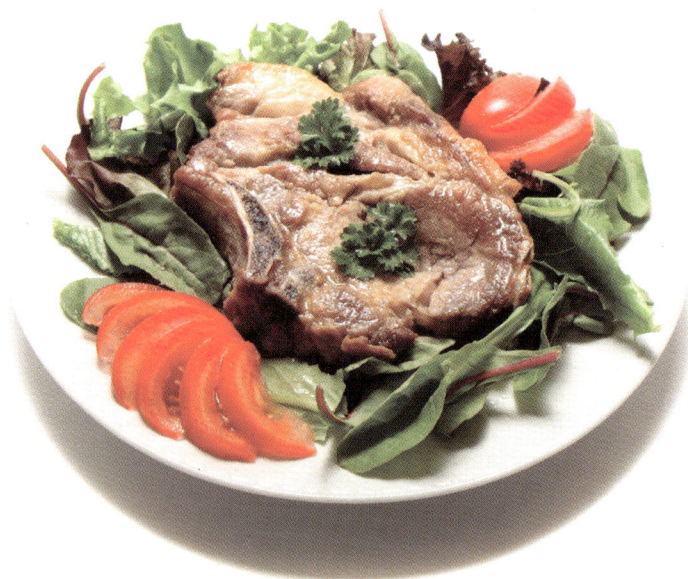

What is important to realise is the source of the food we eat daily. Are we conscious of its nutrition type? Like proteins provide the building blocks and

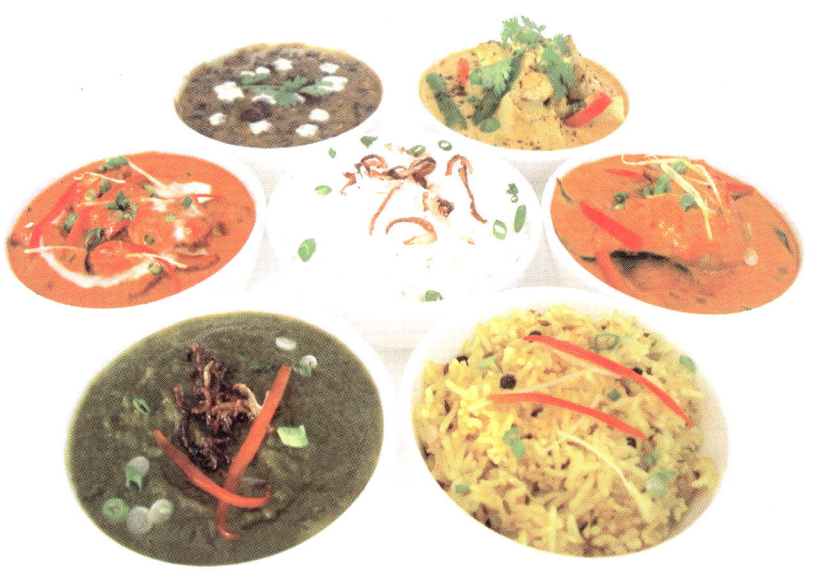

carry on the repairs of the body, carbohydrates supply you with energy and keep you happy. Fats stored in your body are important for the body's warmth. Vitamins and minerals have the privilege of energising your metabolic cycle in order to help your body and mind function normally.

Whatever one consumes as food should be in harmony with nature. Keep the variety of seasonal foods in mind. Those foods may be easily perishable, but they have been produced by nature for that particular geographical area and that climatic condition. Try and tune in with the seasons and your body will be stronger, flexible and healthy.

Fats

Fats are made up of blocks of fatty acids. We eat all kinds of fatty acids without realising what is required and what is in excess. There are three types of fatty acids as mentioned.

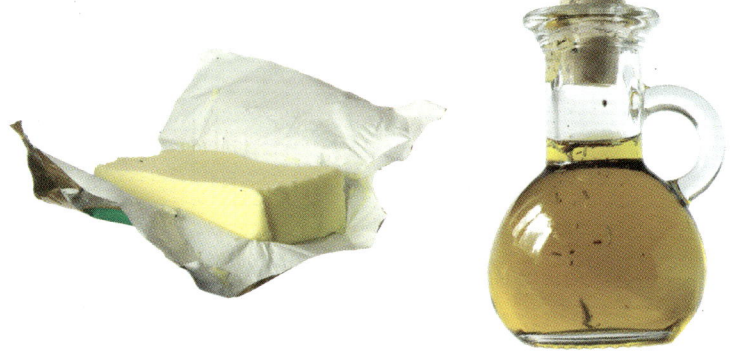

Fatty Acids and Their Sources

Fatty Acids	Composition	Source
Saturated fatty acids (SFA)	Their molecules have no more room for any hydrogen atoms. They are saturated with hydrogen.	Palm oil, coconut oil, dairy products, meats, cocoa butter
Mono unsaturated fatty acids (MUFA)	There is only one bond or area of the fatty acid molecule, which is not saturated with hydrogen atoms.	Olive oil, mustard oil, rapeseed oil, fish, meat
Poly-unsaturated fatty acids (PUFA)	In this fatty acid, more bonds or areas of the molecule can take in hydrogen atoms.	Sunflower oil, soyabean oil, linseed oil, fish

Fatty Acid Composition of Commonly Used Cooking Oils

Oils	Saturated (SFA%)	Monoun-saturated (MUFA%)	Polyun-saturated (PUFA%)
Olive	10	82	8
Canola	6	60	34
Mustard	8	70	22
Soya bean	14	28	58
Sunflower	12	19	69
Groundnut	19	51	30
Coconut	89	7	4
Corn	13	27	60

Try and blend your MUFA and PUFA oils.

Saturated Fats

All saturated fats do not come from animal sources.

- Vegetable oils containing a large amount of saturated fatty acids are coconut and palm oil.
- Consuming less of saturated fat can lower your blood cholesterol.
- Atherosclerosis and thrombosis are the basis of heart attack and strokes. A highly saturated fat diet increases both.

Blended oil is much better than a single variety. This is because taking oil containing too much of polyunsaturated fats can reduce both LDL-cholesterol (bad) and HDL-cholesterol (good cholesterol). Blending oils like olive, mustard (more MUFA) with (more PUFA) oils like sunflower will both decrease your LDL-cholesterol (bad cholesterol) and increase your HDL-cholesterol (good cholesterol). Also, by cutting down on saturated oils in your diet and substituting with more monounsaturated oils you will find an increase in your HDL cholesterol.

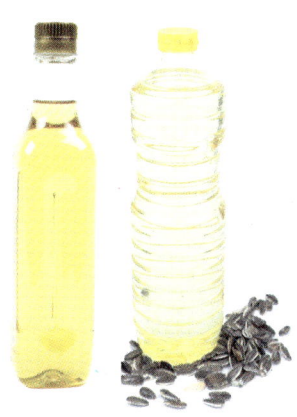

CIS and Trans Fatty Acids

The natural form of the fat molecule is known to be in "cis" form. When this molecule structure is twisted into a different texture, it is said to be in "trans" form and results in the formation of a trans fatty acid. Studies have shown that an increase in LDL-cholesterol (bad cholesterol) increases with increased consumption of trans fatty acids.

Now why is there so much stress on trans and cis fatty acids? It is important to know that changing any oil from liquid into a solid spread (margarine or fat, including the advertised reduced type of fatty acid) involves the adding of hydrogen atoms to the fatty acid molecule.

This is known as "Hydrogenation". Hydrogenated vegetable oils are produced by subjecting vegetable oils to intense heat and pressure in the presence of hydrogen and nickel. This process of hydrogenation results in the formation of trans fatty acids. One must be conscious of the presence of some trans fatty acids in foods with labels – "hydrogenated vegetable oil." Also, the hydro vegetable oil is similar to saturated fat, so try and keep its quantity minimum in your diet.

It is the total amount of fat along with the type of fat consumed every day which has to be considered in your diet (saturated, monounsaturated and polyunsaturated).

Saturated Fatty Acids (SFA)

Saturated fatty acids are to be kept minimal in the diet. These fatty acids increase your LDL-cholesterol. Excessive consumption of foods containing SFA can lead to other diseases besides heart disease. Saturated fatty acids are found in meats, poultry, whole milk dairy products (e.g. milk, cheese, ice cream), etc. Oils which contain a high percentage of saturated fats are coconut and palm.

Monounsaturated Fatty Acids (MUFA)

Monounsaturated fatty acids are in high percentage in olive, mustard, canola and groundnut oil. These oils also contain a good percentage of polyunsaturated fatty acids (PUFA). MUFA helps in lowering LDL-cholesterol (bad cholesterol) and increasing the HDL-cholesterol (good cholesterol).

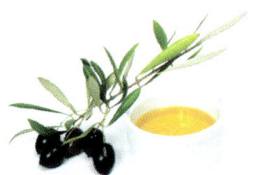
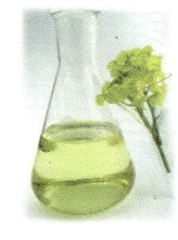

Polyunsaturated Fatty Acids (PUFA)

Polyunsaturated fatty acids are found in a good percentage in canola, mustard, soya bean, sunflower and corn oil. They are found mainly in vegetable oils. The importance of polyunsaturated fatty acids is that it helps skin texture, maintenance and growth.

Eating too much of fat even if it is not of the saturated variety is harmful and can increase your risk for thrombosis (clotting of blood in the arteries).

Avoid reheating and reusing of cooking oils. Reheating can oxidise polyunsaturated fat in your cooking fat, resulting in damage to your blood vessels.

Nuts are high in fat, the exception being of chestnuts. Nuts having monounsaturated and less of saturated fatty acids are hazelnuts, macadamia nuts and almonds. The next good category of nuts (containing polyunsaturated fatty acids) are walnuts and peanuts. Remember that eating of nuts must be limited (not more than one third cup per day or approximately 30 gms per day).

Essential Fatty Acids (EFA)

Fatty acids which cannot be synthesised by the body, but have to be supplied through diet are known as essential fatty acids. Vegetable oils are a good source of EFA.

Essential fatty acids are the precursors of a group of clinically related compounds known as prostaglandins. Prostaglandins play a key role in the body's physiological processes like controlling blood pressure, preventing blood clotting in the arteries, thus avoiding vascular damage to the heart and brain. It also affects women during their menstrual cycles and helps uterine contractions during childbirth.

Prostaglandin
↓
- Causes dilation of blood vessels
- Inhibits platelet aggregation
- Helps in inducing labour
- Increases sensitivity to pain
- Causes fever on infection

Omega Fatty Acids (Omega 3 and Omega 6)

Today Omega fatty acids are the most spoken of, but very few people know what they are all about. Omega 3 fatty acids belong to the unsaturated fatty acids group.

Omega 3

Omega 3 helps in protecting against heart diseases, thrombosis and high blood pressure. It is supposed to lower triglycerides. It is also beneficial in certain inflammatory and autoimmune disorders, e.g. arthritis.

Food Sources of Omega 3

Vegetarian	Non-vegetarian
Flaxseed (oil and seed)	Eggs
Walnuts	Fatty Fish–Hilsa, Surmai, Black Pomfret, Salmon
Oils – Canola (rapeseed) oil Soya bean, Mustard oil	
Green leafy vegetables	
Cereals – Wheat grain, Bajra	
Pulses & Legumes – *Rajmah*, *Lobia*, Urad dal	

Note: Flaxseed oil is easily perishable. It should not be used for cooking. Flaxseed when used, should be ground fresh.

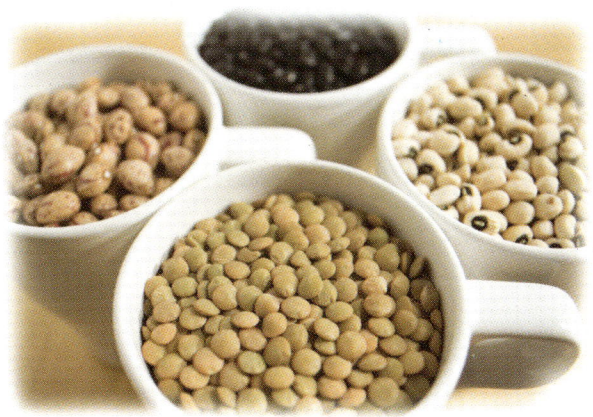

Omega 6

Omega 6 fatty acids belong to the polyunsaturated fatty acid group. More of Omega 6 is consumed in the diet as compared to Omega 3. In fact, one should have more of Omega 3.

Food Sources of Omega 6

Cereals, eggs, baked goodies, whole wheat bread and some vegetable oils.

Total amount of fats to be consumed should be less than 30% of our daily calories.

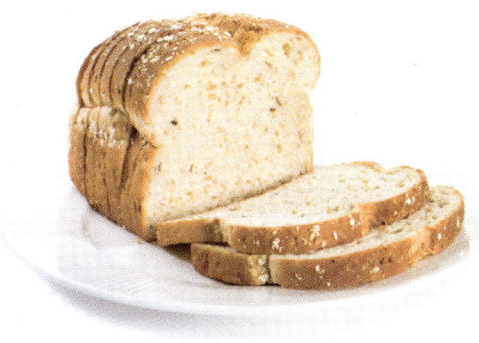
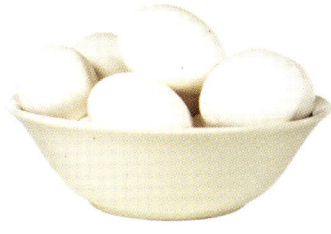

Target the Fat-gram Budget

The average daily dietary fat requirement of a moderately active adult woman is 30 to 40 gms and that of a moderately active adult man is 40 to 60 gms.

An example of 40 grams of fat per day

Breakfast	:	Maximum 5 grams of fat
Mid-morning snack	:	Maximum 3 grams of fat
Lunch	:	Maximum 10 grams of fat
Evening snack	:	Maximum 2 grams of fat
Dinner	:	Maximum 20 grams of fat

Figures are given as estimates only.

The simplest way to save grams of fat is by steadily reducing the quantity of high-fat foods you eat and at the same time increasing your portions of lower-fat or non-fatty foods.

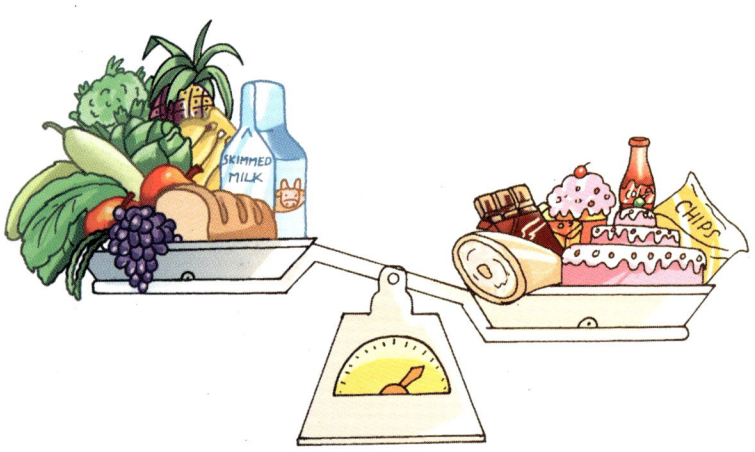

Reducing Grams of Fat in Diet

Carbohydrates

The proportion of carbohydrates consumed throughout the world varies across the globe. Carbohydrates are an important source of energy for the body.

Simple Carbohydrates

Sugars are simple carbohydrates. They can be divided into two types:

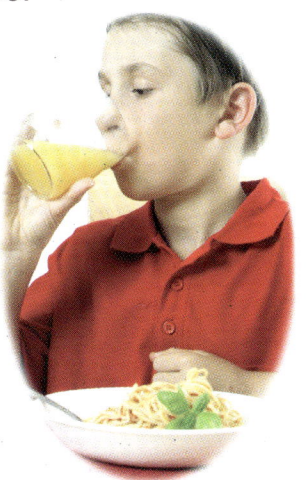

- *Natural sugars:* which are found in natural foods e.g., sugar in vegetables, fruits, etc.
- *Add on sugars:* which have been separated from the natural structure, e.g. table sugar or sugars added in fruit juices, canned products, etc.

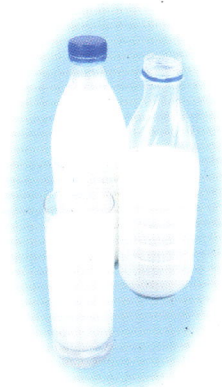

Common Types of Sugars

Type	Name	Source
Fruit sugar	Fructose	Fruits
Milk sugar	Lactose	Milk
Table sugar	Sucrose	Prepared product

Add on sugars which are present, but hidden in breakfast cereals, soft drinks and processed foods should be cut down in your diet. Keep in mind that, honey, brown sugar or white sugar all contain sugar and calories.

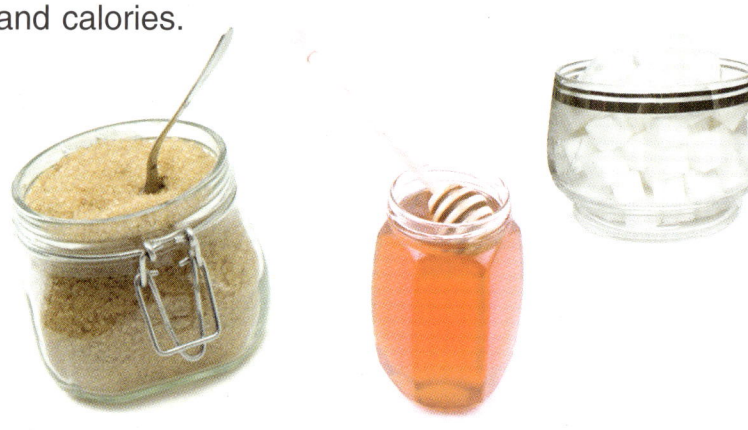

Tips

Drink more water and avoid aerated drinks. Dried fruits can be used to sweeten cakes and other baked products. They are also high in fibre. Tinned fruits or juices should be natural and not with added sweeteners.

Complex Carbohydrates

Starches are the complex carbohydrates. Most of our "eating starches" are consumed in the form of cereal grains, potatoes, beans, peas and other vegetables.

Fibre

The complex carbohydrates group also consists of roughage called "fibre".

Insoluble fibres

They are important for normal bowel functioning. They help in relieving constipation and also lower cholesterol.

Sources

Cereal husk, Esabgol (Psyllium husk), vegetables with skin like potatoes, whole grain cereals, whole wheat bread, brown rice, etc.

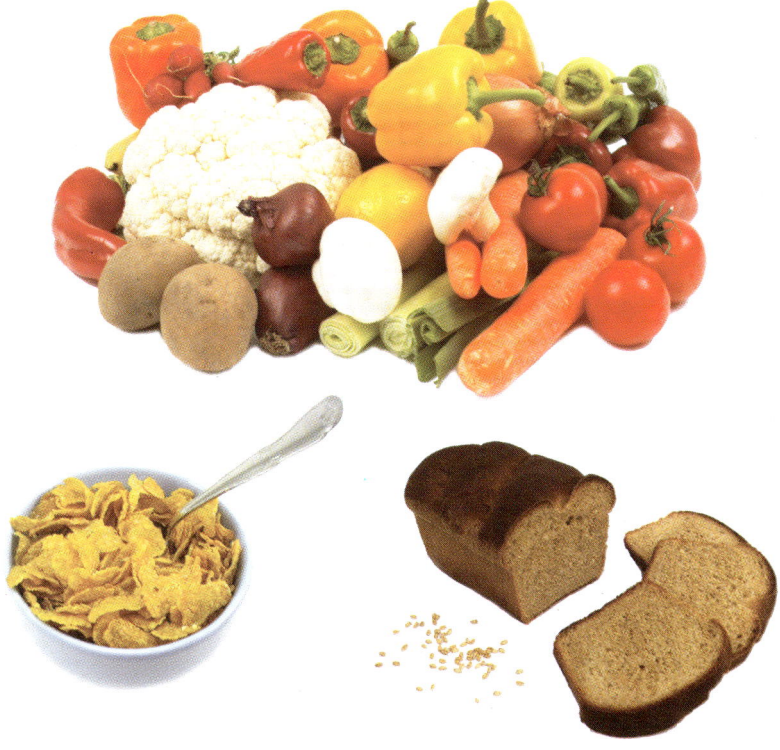

Soluble Fibres

They also help in lowering cholesterol. The theory is that soluble fibres probably bind to the bile acids in the intestine, thus helping in preventing their reabsorption in the body. Soluble fibres also enhance the excretion of cholesterol produced by the liver.

Sources

Oats, fruits (citrus fruits, apple, pear), vegetables and pulses (lentils, beans, chickpea and peas).

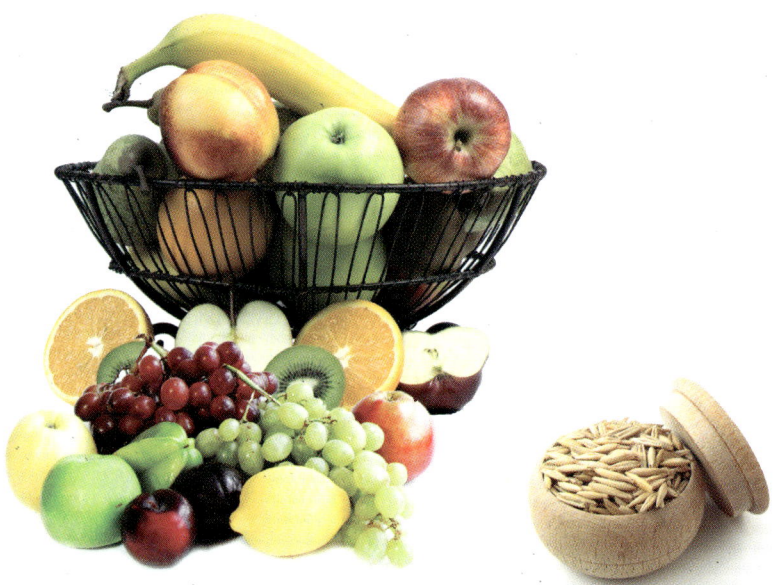

A medium carbohydrate diet should be a part of your meal plan. A high carbohydrate diet, in which the calories are above 60% is not recommended. This is because triglyceride levels are raised and HDL levels are reduced.

Protein

Protein is made up of blocks called amino acids. Your body needs different types of amino acids to keep healthy. There are eight known essential amino acids. Essential amino acids are those which have to be consumed through your diet. Some of the proteins (e.g. meats) that you consume contain all amino acids. Vegetarian sources like vegetables, fruits, grains and nuts are incomplete proteins as they lack one or more amino acids required by the body. These amino acids cannot be manufactured by the body. Vegetarians should be conscious of the fact that to keep themselves healthy they need an assortment of protein containing foods each day. The requirement of protein by the body is about 15-20% of the total calories. The recommended amount of protein for a healthy individual is 0.6 – 0.8 gm/kg body weight.

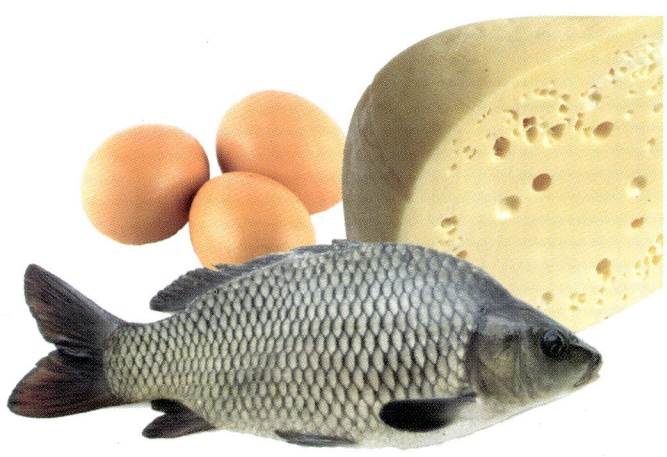

Good Dietary Sources of Proteins

Meats: beef and pork steak

Poultry: chicken breast, turkey breast

Fish: salmon, tuna, crab, lobster, haddock

Dairy products: cheese, milk, yoghurt, tofu, eggs

Lentils: kidney beans

Soyabean: tofu, soya milk, soya granules

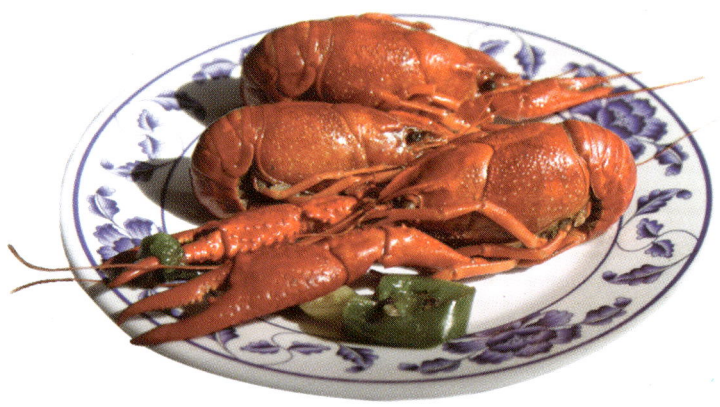

Some Facts about Protein

- Protein is the main building block of our body.
- Protein, next to water is the substance which is found most in our body. It makes up our muscles, ligaments, tendons, nails and hair.
- Protein helps you preserve lean muscle tissues, while you are on a diet to lose fat.

- Protein obtained from animal products (fish, poultry, meat) contain all amino acids. This is called a complete protein.

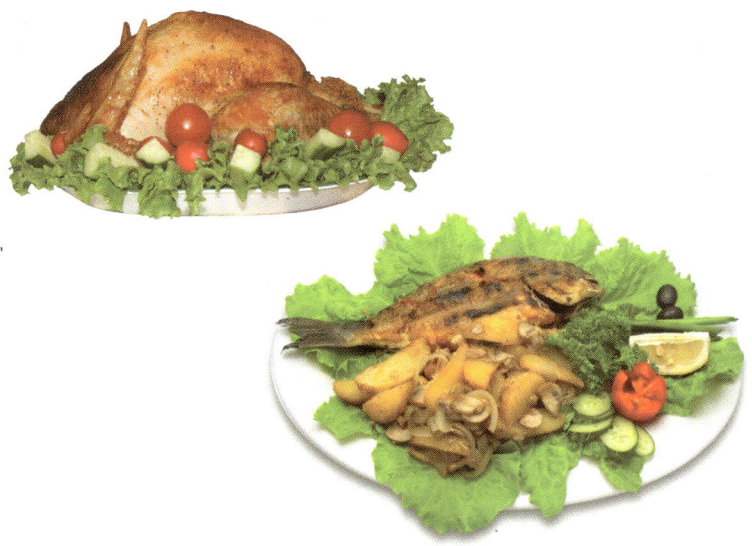

- Protein also helps slowing down the absorption of glucose in the blood stream. This in turn reduces insulin level in your body, making it easier for the body to burn off fat.

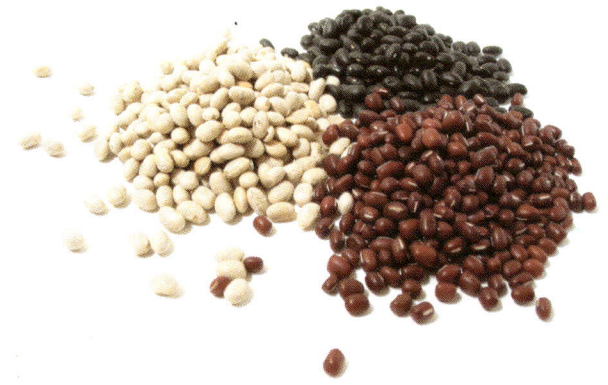

- During protein digestion, certain acids released by the body are usually neutralised with calcium and other buffers in the blood. If one continues consuming high levels of protein, calcium may be depleted from your bones. This may result in osteoporosis (a condition in which bones become weak and are easily broken). In a study, it was seen that women consuming more than 95 gms of protein a day had 20% more broken wrists than those consuming less than 68 gms per day.

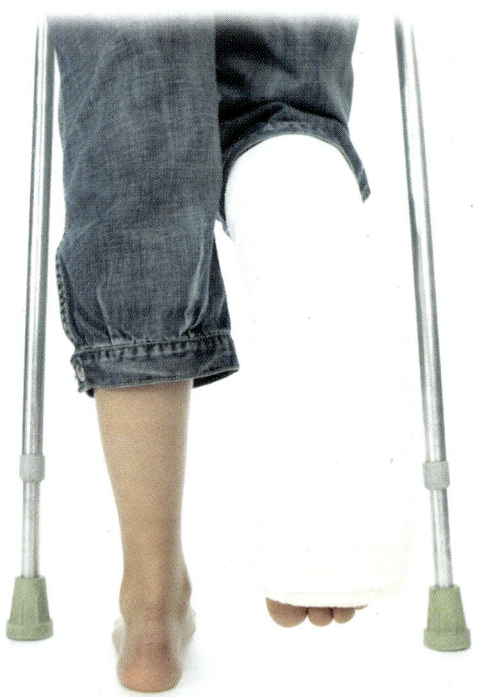

Vegetables

Vegetables are low on the food chain and they support the healthy mid-range pH of the body chemistry. Vegetables are the key sources of the antioxidant vitamins A, C and E. They also contain the supportive co-factors of zinc and the B-complex group of vitamins. The cabbage family vegetables (often called cruciferous) contain amino acids, cysteine and methionine which are antioxidants.

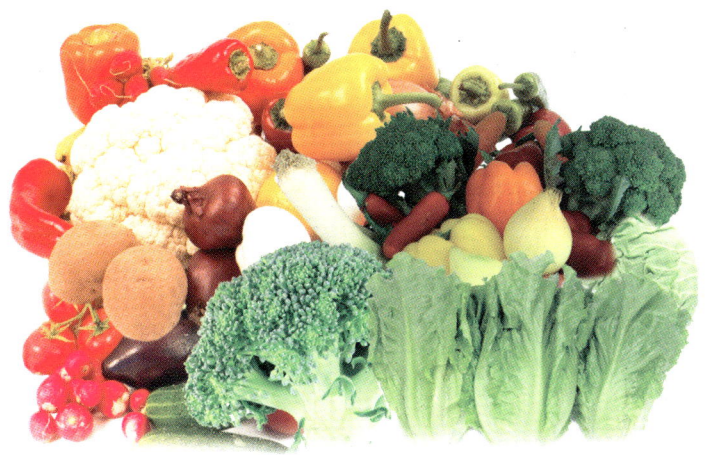

Beans

The bean family contains protease inhibitors which provide protection against certain toxins. Beans are also a good source of the antioxidant vitamins A, C, E, the B complex and zinc co-factor. There are different kinds of beans e.g. lentils, kidney beans, chickpeas, soya beans, lima beans, split beans, pinto and adzuki beans.

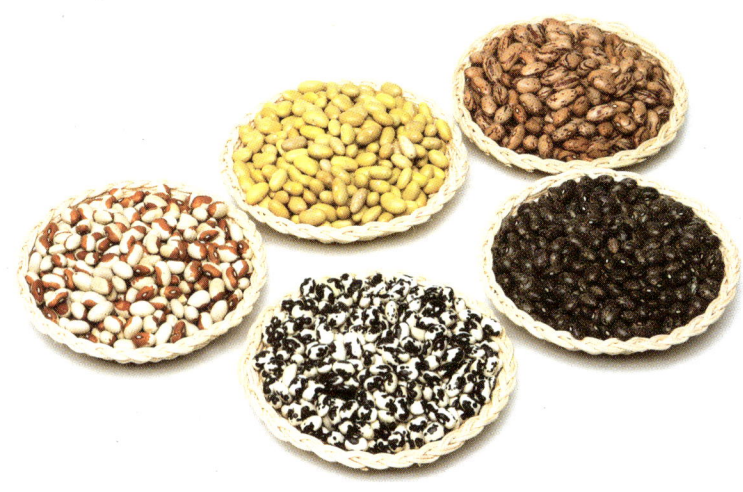

Vitamins and Minerals

Seaweeds

Sea vegetables are full of mineral and trace elements. The calcium content of sea vegetables is especially high. Sea vegetables also contain magnesium, potassium and zinc, which are important for fighting against free radicals.

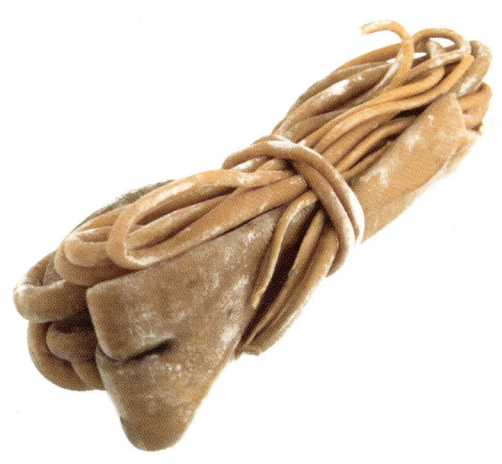

Miso

Miso is a vegetarian source of vitamin B_{12} and is a fermented soya product. Miso's protective power is due to the enzymes it contains.

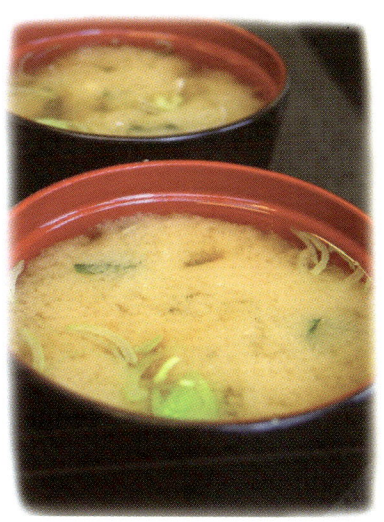

Traditional and Protective Foods

Grains

Grains are important because they provide important nutrients to the body. Grains help to maintain the body's mid-range pH. The bulk of grains helps lessen intestinal transit time, thus helping in the elimination of toxins. Vitamins found in grains have an antioxidant property that helps to eliminate free radicals. The minerals in the grains, act as antioxidant co-factors.

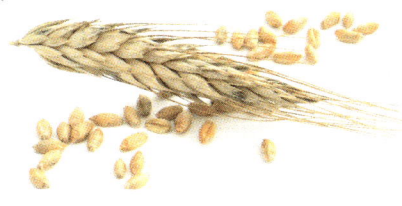
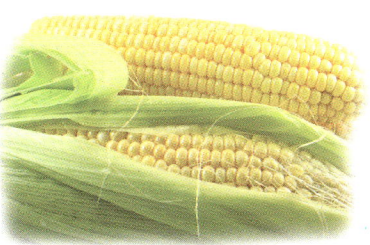

Nutrients Found in Grains

Minerals like calcium, magnesium and vitamin E, etc. are also important nutrients found in grains.

Nuts and Seeds

Nuts and seeds are sources of compact food. They supply protein, B complex vitamins, the antioxidant vitamin E and zinc. Nuts and seeds also contain pectin and phytates, which help eliminate toxins, and in turn reduce free radical formation in the body.

Nuts

Walnuts, brazil nuts, pistachio nuts, pecans, almonds, cashewnuts.

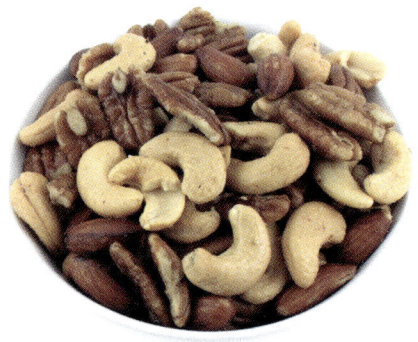

Seeds

Sesame seeds, pumpkin seeds, sunflower seeds.

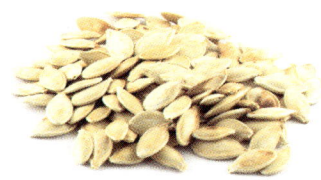

Sprouts

The potential of the B vitamins can increase over 500 percent in the process of growing from seed to sprout. Some of the vegetables that we can sprout regularly and have with our meals are:

Leafy Green Sprouts

Alfalfa, buckwheat, sunflower

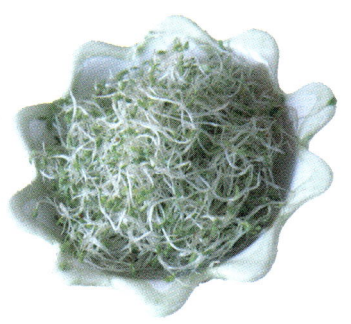

Sprouted Beans

Lentils, *moong*, soya, green peas, *garbanzo*

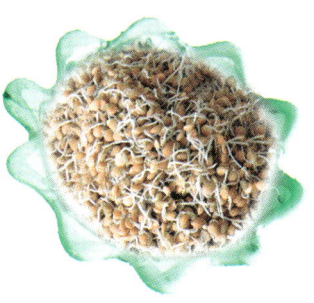

Sprouted Grains

Wheat, rye, barley

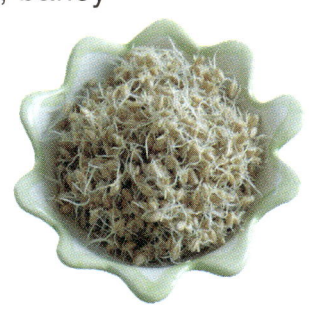

Spices and Condiments

Spices and condiments are commonly used in households for indigestion, flatulence, abdominal cramps and constipation. People in the eastern countries use fenugreek seeds for gout and diabetes, chillies to gain vitamin C, bishop's weed for spasmodic and respiratory disorders. Fennel is often used to relieve flatulence in infants and cloves are used for toothaches. Today turmeric is being considered good for the prevention of cancer.

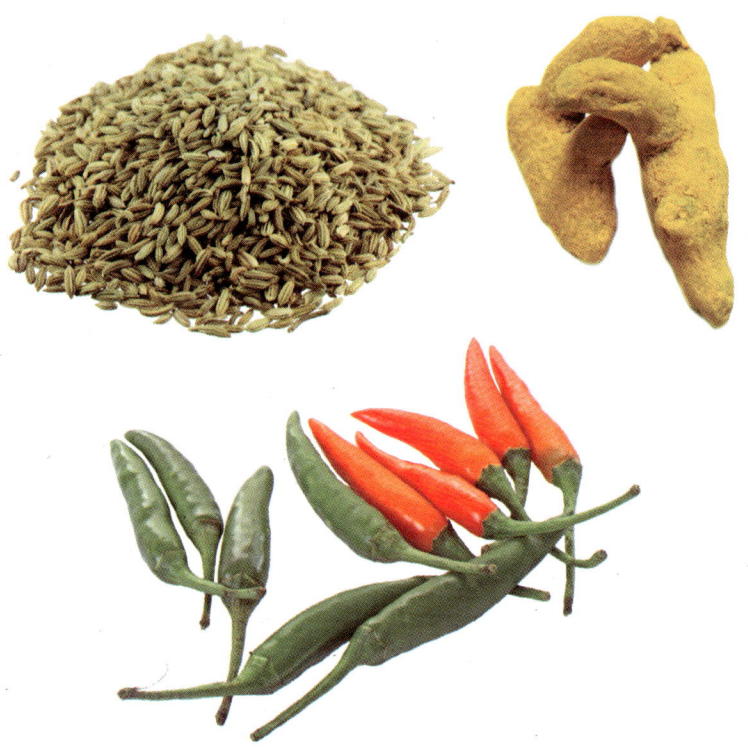

Commonly Used Spices and Condiments

English Name	Indian Name
Bishop's weed	Ajwain
Cardamom (small)	Choti illaichi
Cinnamon	Dalchini
Coriander	Dhania
Chillies	Lal mirchi
Pepper	Kaali mirchi
Basil	Kali tulsi
Asafoetida	Hing
Fennel seed	Saunf
Aniseed	Angrezi saunf
Saffron	Kesar
Fenugreek	Methi
Cumin seed	Jeera
Clove	Laung
Nutmeg	Jaiphal
Mace	Javitri
Bay leaf	Tej patta
Mustard	Sarson
Turmeric	Haldi
Garlic	Lehsan
Ginger	Adrak
Onion	Pyaaz

All the above have some medicinal value, besides being used for flavouring in different kinds of food.

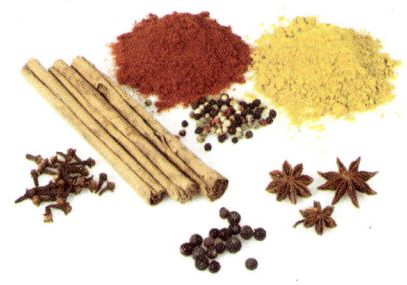

Onion, ginger and garlic are the most commonly grown condiments in many geographical areas of the world. Ginger is known to be valuable against dyspepsia, flatulence, colic and respiratory diseases. Onions are considered good for blood pressure, cough and cold.

Garlic has a variety of therapeutic uses. The range is wide. It extends from helping prevent cardiovascular diseases to cancer to being antibacterial in nature. Garlic is said to lower bad cholesterol in the body and helps reduce clotting in the blood.

Herbs

Through the ages, herbs and medicinal plants have been used by man for healing purposes. As the active principles found in the commonly used herbs are effective in helping prevent certain diseases, they should be used freely in every home.

Commonly Used Herbs

English Name	Indian Name
Dill	Sowa
Celery	Ajmund
Mint	Pudina

Herbs help in counteracting free radicals as they have antioxidant properties. They also help in detoxifying and strengthening your immune system. Some of the commonly used herbs are - dill (*sowa*), celery (*ajmund*), mint (*pudina*), etc.

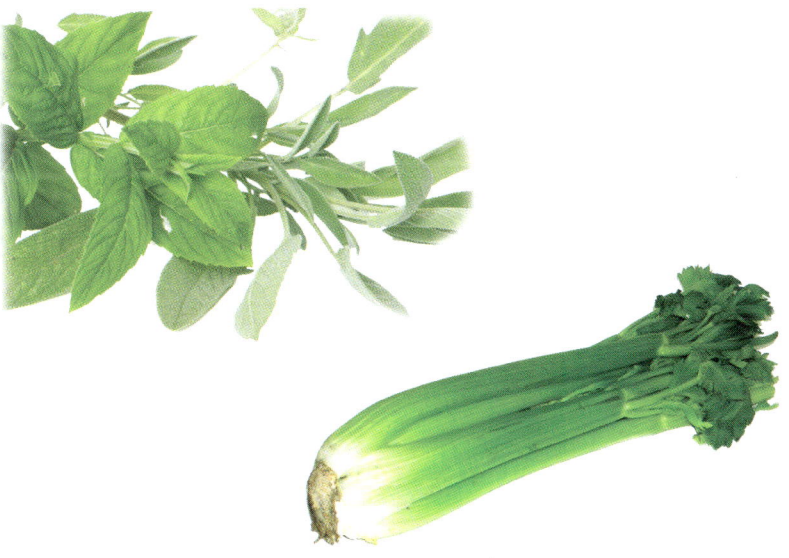

High Nutrient Sea Vegetables

Algae have multiple nutrients and free radical fighting antioxidants and antioxidant enzymes.

Algae contain vitamin B, Beta-carotene, and minerals including iron and magnesium. They also contain proteins which are available as neuropeptides which help fortify the neuro transmission. Chlorophyll present in the algae fights free radicals.

Vitamins, Minerals and Medication

Vitamins help in the normal functioning of the body. They are also essential for scavenging free radicals from the body and are important for fighting diseases. Commonly used medication often depletes the body of vitamins and minerals.

Depleted Vitamins and Minerals due to Certain Medications

Medication	Depleted Vitamins and Minerals
Alcohol	Magnesium, Vitamin B complex, Vitamin C, D, E and K
Antibiotics	Vitamin B and K
Anti-Inflammatories	Vitamin C, Folic Acid, Iron
Antihistamines	Vitamin C
Antihypertensives	Calcium, Potassium, Magnesium, Vitamin B, Folic acid
Aspirin	Vitamin A and B, Calcium, Folic acid, Iron, potassium
Caffeine	Potassium, Vitamin B, Zinc
Diuretics	Calcium, Iodine, Magnesium, Potassium, Vitamin C, Zinc
Estrogen	Vitamin B_6, Folic acid
Laxatives	Vitamin A, D & K, Potassium, other minerals

3 *Keep Your Palate Under Control*

All tasty food may not be helpful for your well-being. Be conscious of what you eat. Once in a while, letting the senses rule the mind is fine. At the same time remember, its you who has to keep the balance!

Salt

It is estimated that 1 gm of salt contains 2.4 gms of sodium. If the average daily salt intake is reduced to about one-third by people, it would help prevent blood pressure and strokes. The commonly used salt products we consume without being conscious are:

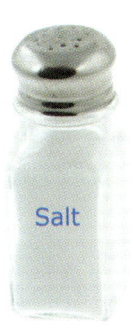

Salt

- Butter
- Cornflakes
- All breads
- Pickles
- Processed foods
- Soups and sauces
- Meats like bacon
- Canned and processed food
- Snacks (*pakoras*, *samosas*, wafers, chips)

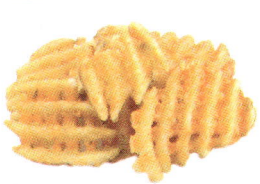

Most foods eaten contain much more salt than is required by our body. Try and pick up processed (canned and packed) food with less sodium and sweet content. Do read the labels on the food that you pick from your stores.

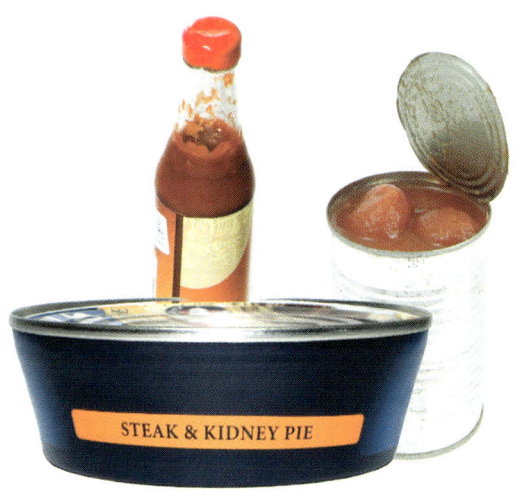

Points to Remember

- Avoid adding extra salt when cooking or eating.
- If hypertensive, or otherwise try using less salt.
- Season more with spices and herbs.
- To add flavour and not miss salt, you can also use vinegar, lemon and wines for cooking.

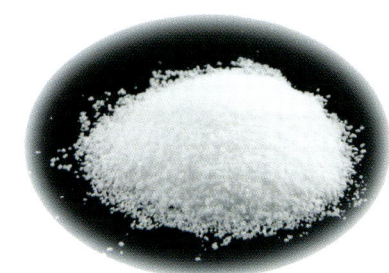

- Broil, grill, bake or steam food without adding salt or fat. Use nonstick pans or cookware. Microwave if essential.

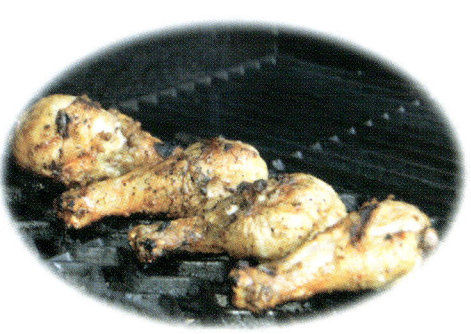

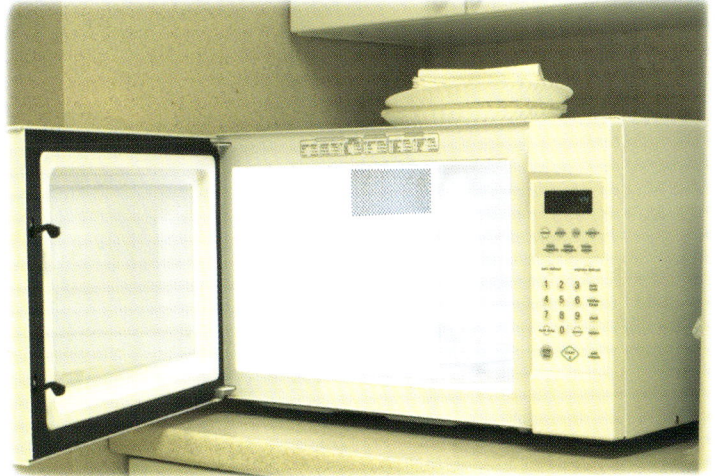

Sugar

It appears that the calories simply get replaced by other foods. It has also been found that sweets (even artificial ones) stimulate an appetite for fats in some people.

Refined white sugar – sucrose – tops the list of "empty calories", along with its counterparts – corn syrup, brown sugar, dextrose, fructose, maltose and cane syrup. It makes sense to moderate your consumption of sweeteners and of highly sweetened foods – especially when they are eaten with highly fatty foods.

If your tight schedule often makes it necessary for you to eat meals and snacks away from home, make healthy choices. Add more fresh salads, grain/lasagna, whole wheat bread, chapati, brown rice, baked or boiled potato and lot of vegetables to your diet.

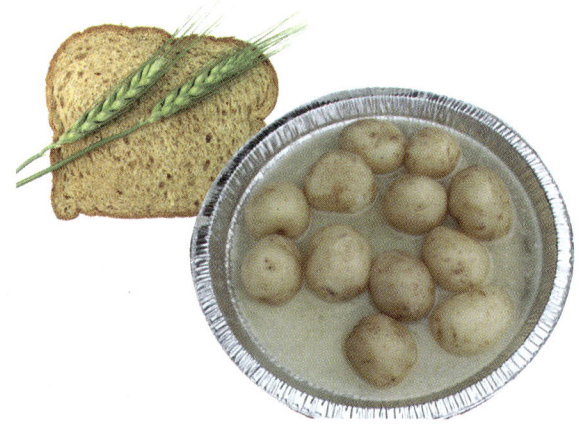

Dairy Products

Milk and its products should be consumed in moderate quantity (approximately not more than 500 gms/day). Low fat or skimmed milk should be preferably consumed.

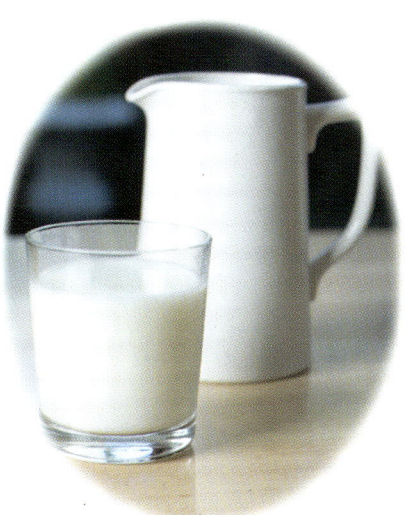

Cheese

Cheese has a high fat content, two-third of which is likely to be saturated. When eating cottage cheese one must realise that a certain amount of saturated fat is present. So don't binge too much on dairy products.

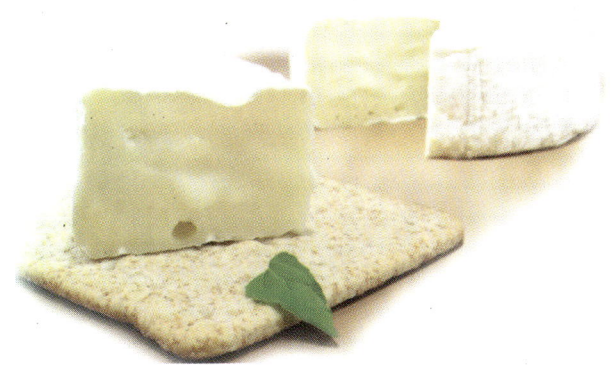

Alcohol and Snacking

The lowest risk is for those who drink one or two small drinks/day (30ml/daily). The risk shoots up on 4 drinks/day. The recommended safe drinking limit is lower for women than men. As a woman's body contains less water than a man, it takes less alcohol in a woman to reach a harmful concentration.

One unit of alcohol is obtained as:
- 25 ml of whisky or other spirits
- 125 ml of a glass of wine
- 50 ml of Martini or Sherry (fortified wine)

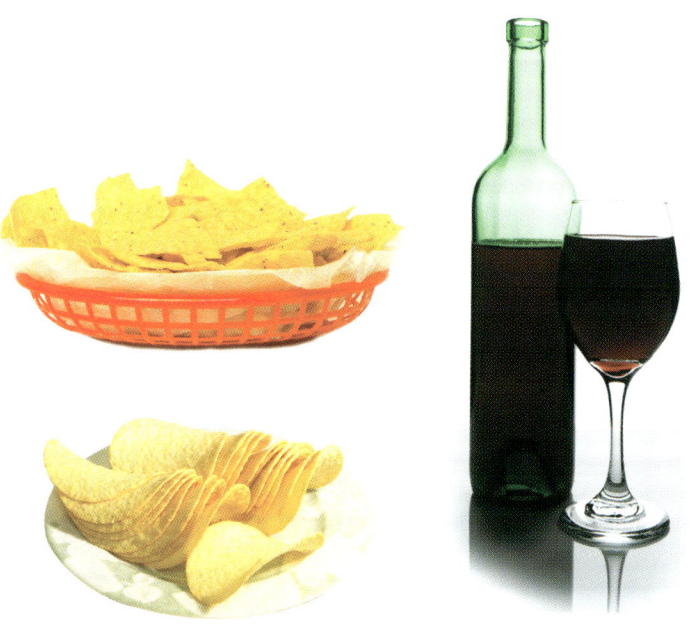

Points to Remember

- One peg of whisky/rum/vodka (approx. 40 ml) is about 105 calories. A glass of wine contains 85-135 calories.
- Alcohol, is a source of empty calories (i.e. it does not contain minerals and vitamins). It adds fat to the body. It provides higher calories than any other food, e.g. carbohydrates and proteins.
- Alcohol is also a great appetiser.

Most people like to snack while drinking alcoholic beverages. One must remember that along with carbohydrates (wafers, potato fries, cheeslings, etc.) you take in alcohol calories as well. Try and keep to salads (without high fat dressings) or small amounts of nuts (without too much salt or oil), when consuming alcohol.

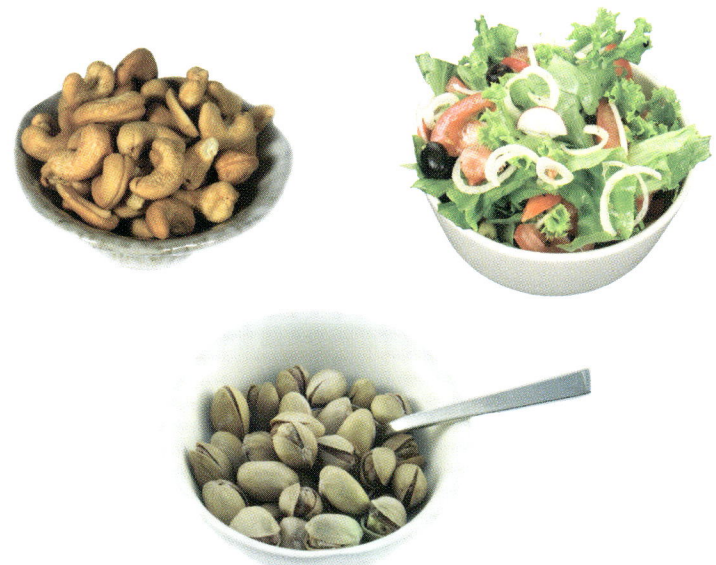

4 A Healthy Meal Plan

Water

Water contains no carbohydrates, proteins or fats. It possesses no calories. It is the most overlooked component in nutrition.

Water : Crucial for Survival

- Water stabilises the body temperature.
- It helps transport nutrients throughout the body.
- It excretes waste products.
- It is a part of blood and other body fluids.
- Water is essential for joint lubrication.

Daily Requirement

- 2.0 – 2.5 litres of water is required / day. In warm weather or while exercising you need more water.

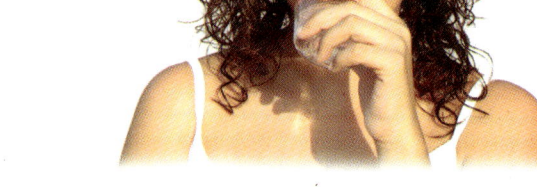

Water is Lost by the Body Daily

- As urine
- From the lungs
- As faeces
- Through the skin

Water is Provided

- More by foods, such as fruits or vegetables.
- Other foods like pastries, cakes, butter provide little water.
- Food when broken down for energy also provides water.

Drinks that Hydrate Your Body

- Water
- Fruit juice
- Skimmed milk
- Herbal teas

Drinks that Dehydrate Your Body

- Caffeinated drink
- Coffee
- Tea
- Colas
- Certain energy drinks
- Alcohol

Drinks or fruit juices high in sugar slow down water absorption from your stomach.

The Body and Energy

60-75% of your total daily energy spent is used for keeping you alive. It is also known as the *resting metabolic rate* and is the number of calories you use, if you rest in the bed the whole day. It does not give your ideal calorie intake.

Approximately 10% of the total daily energy spent is used for digesting your foods.

15-30% of the total daily energy is used for physical activity.

Total Daily Energy (100%)

- Resting metabolic rate (60-75% energy)
  - Heart beat and circulation
  - Breathing
  - Repair of tissues
- Eating food (10% energy)
  - Eating and digesting food
  - Absorbing nutrients
- Physical activity (15-30% energy)

To Calculate Your Resting Metabolic Rate (RMR)

Multiply your weight in *lbs* by 10 (*lbs* x 10)

(1 *lb* = 0.45 kg)

If you weigh 120 *lb* your RMR will be approximately 1200 calories.

Glycaemic Index

Glycaemic index is a ranking of carbohydrates on a scale of 0 to 100, based on their immediate effect on blood sugar after eating.

Foods with a high glycaemic index   (70+)
Foods with a medium glycaemic index   (55 to 69)
Foods with a low glycaemic index   (55 or less)

Low glycaemic index has been shown to help improve glucose and lipid levels in people with diabetes (both Type I and Type II). They do not promote fat storage. Foods with low glycaemic index help control excessive appetite, delay hunger thereby helping in weight control.

Foods with High Glycaemic Index

White bread, potatoes, juices, dates, corn flakes and glucose.

Foods with Intermediate Glycaemic Index

Brown bread, popcorn, white rice, sweet corn, cheese pizza, canned peaches, instant oatmeal, fresh pineapple.

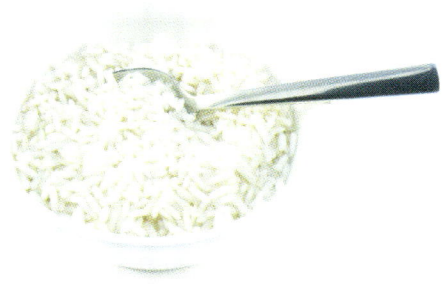

Foods with Low Glycaemic Index

Vegetables, fruits, oats, whole wheat bread, pasta, parboiled rice, barley, fat free or skimmed milk and yogurt.

Organic Food

Organic food are those which are produced without the use of artificial pesticides, herbicides or any synthetic products. They may be produced or grown in a farm, home or bought from a store.

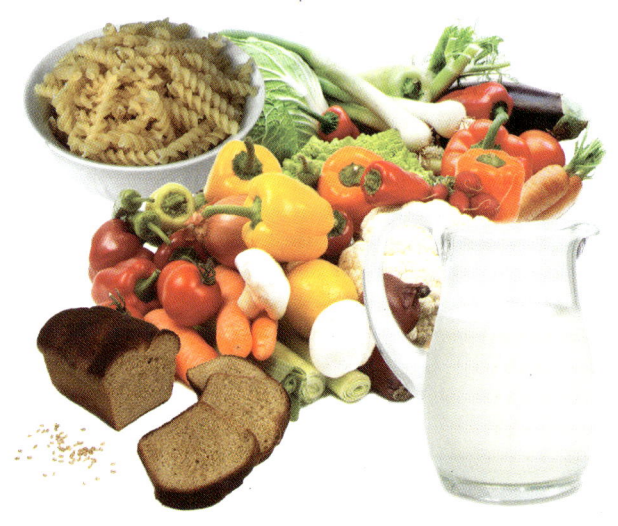

Organic foods can be fresh or frozen. Fresh foods like vegetables and fruits are seasonal and perishable. They are best consumed during the months that they are grown in. This is also in regard to their nutrient value. Therefore organic foods can be defined as products grown without extensive use of synthetic chemicals and which are normally seasonal products.

Processed foods can also be organic though they may or may not be seasonal. These foods are processed without artificial methods, e.g. no chemical ripening (with ethylene) or no food irradiation.

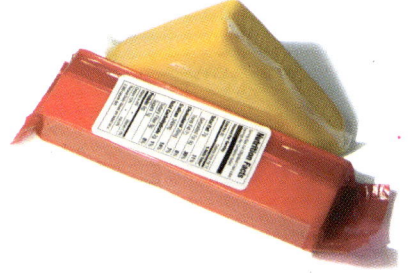

Fibre

Fibre helps in slowing down absorption of glucose in the blood. Average fibre intake/day should be around 40 gms for men and 25 gms for women. Fibre is the indigestible cellulose material in grains, vegetables and fruits. *Choker atta*, i.e. the unrefined *atta*, is important for the body's metabolism.

Also fibre in foods (if substituted for fatty foods) helps reduce cholesterol and triglycerides in the body.

Balanced Nutritive Plan

Foods to Enjoy Regularly	Foods to Enjoy in Moderation	Foods to be Avoided
Cereal Parboiled rice, missi roti, preparation of *kuttu ka atta*, *dalia*, chapati, whole grain cereal, brown bread, whole wheat bread Oatmeal, low sugar breakfast cereal, whole wheat pasta, brown rice, low sugar muesli (no nuts, coconut). **Vegetables** Fresh, frozen, tinned	**Cereal** Vermicelli (*sevian*), rice flakes (*chidwah*), *khichri*, home baked goods using unsaturated oil **Milk and Milk Products** Skimmed milk Cottage cheese Very low fat yoghurt Very low fat ice cream Fat free cheese Peanut butter **Nuts** Chestnuts Almonds	**Cereal** *naan*, *bhature*, puris, cereals with nuts, coconut **Milk and Milk Products** Whole milk, Cream Coffee whitener Full fat yoghurt Full fat cheese Ice cream Butter, cheese (like parmesan and cheddar). **Cooking Fats & Oils** **Nuts** Cashewnuts **All Fatty Sauces and Dressings** Mayonnaise, Egg yolk, Fat dripping, etc **Meat Products** Pie, salami burger, mutton, meats

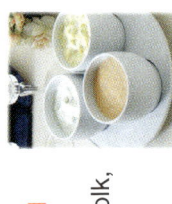
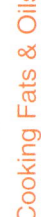
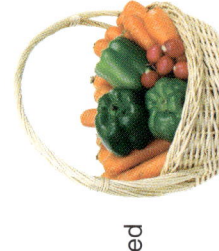

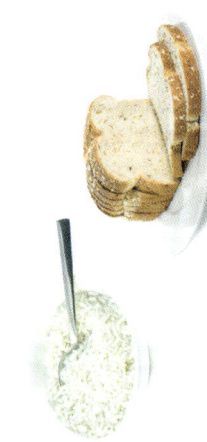

Bakery and Confectionery
Cake, biscuits, pastries, cheese biscuits, cream crackers, croissants, Indian sweets, *ladoo, burfi*, etc.
Muffins, doughnuts, biscuits

Vegetables cooked in oil or butter

Fast Food
Deep fried chips, burger, hot dogs, pizzas, *chole bhature, dosa* with coconut chutney, *samosa, pakora*

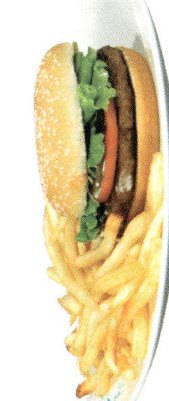

Dessert
Toffee apples, banana fritters, *halwas*

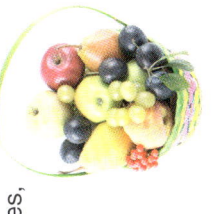

Fruits
Mangoes, grapes, olives, avocados, bananas
Unsweetened Tinned

Others
Chocolate spread
Grilled food

Meat and Meat Products
Skinless chicken
Turkey breast
Fish
Shell fish

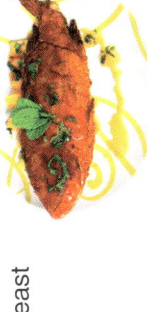

Fried Foods
Pancakes, *parantha* (minimum oil) roast potato, chips (suitable less oil)

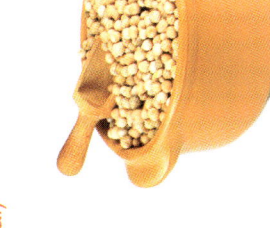

Fruits
Dried, natural or tinned

Salads

Egg white

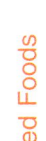

Soya products
Tofu, Quern

Beans
Peas, Chickpea

Fatless cake

Lentils (*Dal*)

A Few Lines on...

Gout

Gout is a disease which is caused by low enzymatic levels of purine metabolism or high levels of uric acid product. Uric acid is the metabolic end product of proteins (i.e. purine nucleic acids). Some purines are made by our body while some are consumed through the foods we eat. High levels of uric acid can cause formation of crystals in the joints and cartilage of the body.

Reducing the amount of purines in protein helps in the reduction of uric acid.

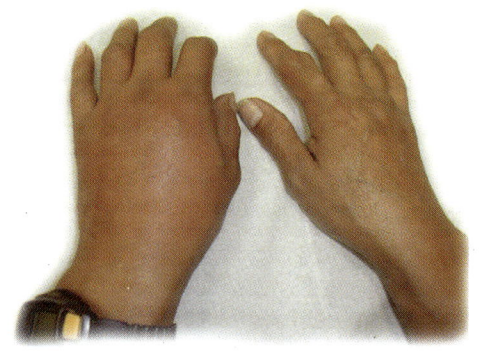

Swollen Hands caused by Gout

Kidney (Oxalate) Stones

Oxalic acid in the course of being processed in the body combines with the salts like calcium to form salts of calcium oxalates. It can precipitate in crystalline form as stones in the kidney. Oxalate stones are also found in the bladder.

Sources of Food with High Oxalic Acid

Lettuce, eggplant, sweet potato, spinach, radish, parsley, cabbage, broccoli, garlic, etc.

People with a renal stone or bladder stone should avoid these or have them less in their diet.

Some Foods with Different Purine Levels

High level purines	Moderate level purines	Low level purines
Fish – sardine cod, trout	*Meat* – beef, pork	Grains Milk products Sugar
Poultry – turkey	*Sea food* – crab, lobster, oyster	Green vegetables
Organ – liver, kidney	*Poultry* – chicken, duck	Eggs
	Kidney beans and lentils	Bread
Other sources – alcohol	*Vegetables* – spinach, mushrooms	Coffee

Malnutrition

It is a complex condition resulting from an imbalance between the body's need and intake of nutrients. It can involve deficiencies of proteins, micronutrients (vitamins and minerals). It can also lead to toxicity dependency or obesity.

Causes of Malnutrition

Undernutrition: Results from inadequate intake of nutrients (during an illness) or an imbalanced diet.

Overnutrition: Results from overeating (mainly wrong types of food), insufficient exercise and also overprescription of the fad therapeutic diets. This leads to excess intake of vitamins (toxicity) and deficiency of minerals. A person may be overweight, but due to improper nutrition can be malnourished.

Fad Diets: Yo-yo dieting is not recommended. Low calorie diets cannot sustain the body for long and result in vitamin, mineral and protein deficiencies. These deficiencies can thereby result in serious metabolic disorders.

Drug or alcohol dependency often leads to wrong eating habits. Absorption and metabolism of nutrients due to alcohol is impaired. Alcohol consumers with unhealthy food habits often gain weight. Hard liquor consumers are often known to suffer from deficiencies of thiamine, calcium, magnesium, zinc and other nutrients.

Some Common Signs of Malnutrition

Swollen or bleeding gums

Dry and scaly skin

Pigmentation of hair

Spooned nails

Painful bones and joints

Malnutrition in Children

Inadequate intake of protein, (to build muscles and keep the body healthy) calories (for energy), iron (for proper functioning of blood cells), vitamins and minerals are the main causes of malnutrition in children.

The body's requirements for micronutrients is essential, especially in the growing stages and geriatric phase (old age). Micronutrients needed are Vitamins A, B, C, folate zinc, calcium, iron and iodine.

Some Common Deficiency Diseases

Goitre (Enlarged thyroid gland): Due to iodine deficiency.

Vitamin A deficiency: Leading cause of *(preventable)* blindness in children.

Anaemia: It leads to low red blood cells count. Anaemia causes tiredness, can affect brain functioning and cause cardiac death in severe cases.

Treatment of these diseases is through fortified foods and supplements. If the amount of food is not enough the body does not receive energy. In children there is weight loss due to lack of muscle mass. Malnourished children have disproportionately large abdomen, little muscle and inadequate fat stores. They also have a high incidence of diseases as the body is not well-equipped to fight infection.

Food Labels and Good Nutrition

How to Read Food Labels

The information given to you on the back of your food packet or tin gives the nutritional quality of the product you are buying.

Calories: Calories are shown either as "K calories", "kilojoules" or "energy". They are listed per serving or per 100 gm. Food can be of low calorie, but still have refined sugar or fat.

Protein: Protein present is often in small amounts. Check for animal or vegetable sources.

Carbohydrates: Carbohydrates are sometime subdivided into sugars or starches. So they are read as "refined" and "complex" carbohydrates. Complex carbohydrates should be preferred. Remember that sugar provides energy, but has little nutritional value.

Fat: All fat is fattening.

- You should be careful about the total amount of the fat consumed.
- Avoid fat which is saturated.
- Unsaturated fat is equally fattening but is a healthier choice.

  Note : Reduced fat foods can often contain upto 40% of fat.

Strike a Balance For Good Nutrition

- Do not keep counting calories.
- Drink a lot of water.
- Strike a balance in selecting different types of food for your plate.
- See that they are right in proportion.
- Get your calories
  - More from complex carbohydrates
  - Fewer from fat
- Eat in moderation

Be Totally Fit: Exercise and Eat Right

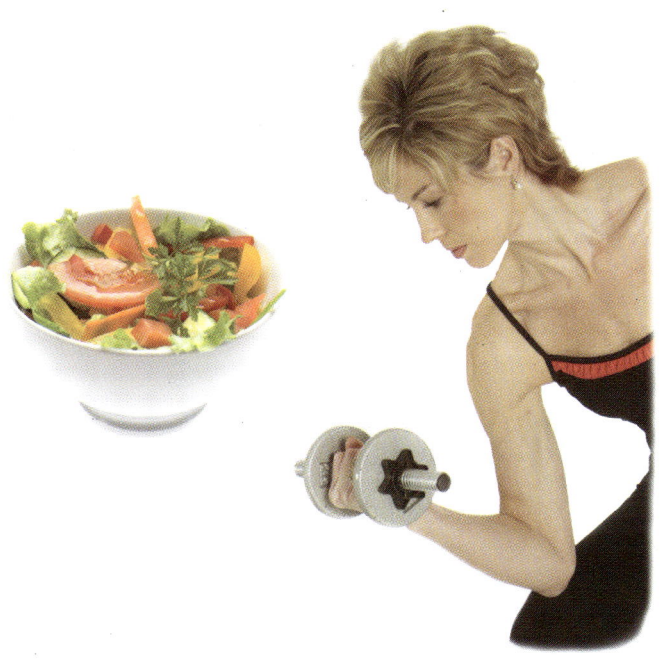

Nutrients In Your Food Blocks

Nutrients	Vegetables	Other Natural Sources	Action of Vegetables
Vitamin A	Carrots, corn, green beans, tomato, kale, all dark green leafy greens, squash, zucchini, broccoli	Fish, liver oils, mango, apricots, milk and milk products	Antioxidant, defends against infection, helps in keeping the skin healthy. Aids in better vision.
B Complex	All vegetables		Good antioxidant cofactor, helps in fortifying immune system.
Vitamin C	All green vegetables, potato, red peppers, green chillies, tomato	Orange, raspberry, fruit juices, cranberry, grape, sweet potato	Antioxidant, helps increase immunity, defends against infection. Helps wound healing. Prevents scurvy.
Vitamin D	Sunlight	Fortified milk and cereals, egg yolk, fish (salmon, tuna), watermelon	Promotes healthy bones and strong teeth. Helps prevent osteoporosis.
Vitamin E	All leafy greens	Vegetable oil, sunflower seeds, nuts, fish, eggs, chicken liver	Antioxidant, helps in maintaining healthy skin and aids in circulation. Helps in healing of the skin.
Calcium	All green vegetables, broccoli, etc.	Dairy products, milk, cheese, tofu, fish, almonds, wheat germ	Builds bones, blocks absorption of certain toxins. Helps reduce heart burn, prevents blood clotting and maintains pH balance.
Magnesium	All vegetables	Nuts (almond, cashews), whole grains, tofu, beans, lentils, apples, milk, cheese, chicken, yogurt	Maintains pH balance, aids in nerve and muscle function. Helps in bone and tooth formation, converts blood sugar into energy.
Sulphur	All cabbage family		Helps repair free radical damage to DNA

Mineral	Sources	Functions
Potassium	All vegetables	...nerve impulse and muscle contraction, regulates heart beat and decreases the risk of high BP.
Fibre	All vegetables	Binds and helps the body to get rid of toxins.
Zinc	Sea vegetables	Helps in healing of wounds, immune booster, improves insulin levels, helps in building healthy scalp and hair. Regulates metabolism of male hormone.
Iron	Vegetables, spinach, peas, beans	Prevents anaemia. Aids growth. Provides energy, prevents fatigue. Helps enhance immune system.
Selenium	Broccoli, mushroom, garlic	Antioxidant protecting damage by free radicals. Vitamin E and selenium work together to fight diseases like heart disease and cancer.
Iodine	Vegetables (grown in iodine rich soil), salt water fish	Helps in healthy thyroid function, promotes proper growth, weight loss and efficient body metabolism. Helps in having healthy nails, skin and hair.
Chromium	Broccoli, potato, peas, legumes	Improves glucose tolerance. Essential for proper growth and body function. Nutrient for overall health and growth.
Copper	Peas, garlic, mushroom, potato	Immunity booster, helps in the manufacture of enzymes, coating of nerve fibres and collagen.

The B Complex Group

Nutrients	Vegetables	Other Natural Sources	Action of Vegetables
Folic Acid	Spinach, asparagus, vegetables	Fortified foods	Protects against birth defects, helps prevent cardiovascular and other diseases.
Riboflavin (B_2)	Green leafy vegetables, spinach, broccoli, mushrooms.	Milk, yogurt, cheese, bread, cereals, liver	Helps in growth and reproduction, antioxidant, alleviates fatigue, important for nerve function and metabolism.
Niacin (B_3)	Green leafy vegetables, spinach, broccoli, mushrooms	Milk, cheese, poultry, wheat germ, brown rice, enriched bread, cereals, dates, figs, prunes, etc.	Important for preventing heart diseases, promotes healthy body metabolism. Helps in increasing good cholesterol, aids in preventing anxiety.
Pyridoxin (B_6)	Vegetables	Fruits, fortified cereals, meat, poultry, fish	Maintains healthy immune system, helps maintain normal blood sugar, normal nerve conduction, and prevents neuropathy.
Cobalamin (B_{12})	Green leafy vegetables, spinach, broccoli, mushrooms	Lamb, fish, (trout, sardine), eggs, milk, and milk products, organ meats.	Helps prevent anaemia, helps in maintaining immunity.

Myths and Fact File

Myth

Ghee, butter and lot of cream in milk is healthy.

Fact

All saturated fat like ghee, butter and cream are detrimental to health. Saturated fat both in vegetarian and non-vegetarian form, should be less than 7% of our diet (of 30% total fat consumed as part of the calories in a day).

Myth

Crash dieting is a good way to lose weight quickly.

Fact

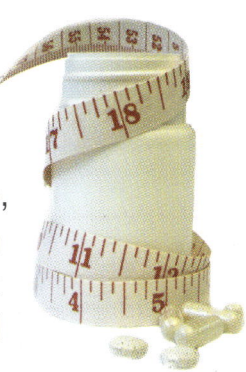

Crash dieting is not good for general health. One must lose weight slowly (not more than ½ kg a week). Otherwise, nutrition imbalance can occur. On reaching the ideal weight, maintain it through proper nutritional diet and regular exercise. Yo-yo dieting makes you put on more weight.

Myth

Drinking lot of tea or juices in the day will help me fulfil the requirements of fluids.

Fact

Tea and juices are to be taken in measured quantities. Water the elixir of health is required in large quantities to clean your body of wastes and toxins.

Myth

Pickles are harmless. I can have them regularly with all my meals.

Fact

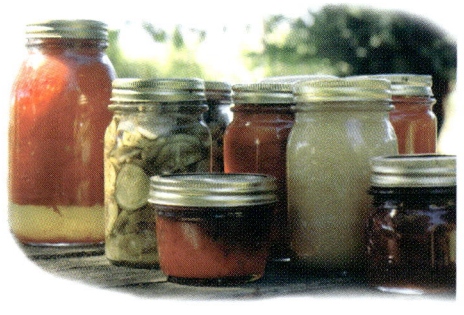

Be conscious of the fact that pickles are preserved in lot of oil and salt, both of which should be taken in less amount. Fresh pickle made in lemon juice with less salt, can be consumed regularly.